Get your head straight.

John Kim MA, MFT

This book is designed for people who would rather be doing muscle ups.

There are no chapters in this book. There are only two sections, Micro and Macro.

Micro is the candy, quick mental techniques, tips, and exercises that you can start applying today. They are a combination of concepts found in sports psychology as well as my own that I have come up with throughout my CrossFit journey. I have put them through a psychobabble filter so that I can present them to you in plain English.

Macro is the protein, the reason I wrote this book. It's my take on mental blocks and how to dissolve them. As a fellow CrossFitter, I would like to say "crush", but rewiring your mind involves a process, not a button. I hang my theory on five truths.

Truth One: I believe CrossFit is about stories and the power behind them. I believe CrossFit is about rebuilding ourselves through others. I practice this philosophy online with my public practice - running therapeutic groups via webcam. It's what drew me to CrossFit and keeps me there. The core beliefs of CrossFit line up with my own which is why I wrote this book. Mind/Set is not only an approach, it is an invitation to process your CrossFit journey with other CrossFitters around the world.

So who am I and how am I qualified to discuss the mental aspect of athletic performance?

I am not a fire breather. I do not have a sub 3 minute Fran. I am just your average John. I CrossFit four times a week. I try to eat Paleo but I struggle daily with my sweet tooth. I have addictive tendencies. I have false beliefs. I am obsessive. I chase the Leaderboard. I internalize. And, I hate overhead squats.

I am also a Marriage Family Therapist. I have worked with addicts and eating disorder patients in both residential and outpatient settings. I have facilitated groups, family, and individual sessions, and spearheaded a family support program for a nonprofit alcohol and drug abuse organization in Los Angeles.

About two years ago, I left the 9 to 5 and started a blog. Today, I use this blog as a therapeutic tool to help people with their relationships, addictions, and self esteem. I help them build new containers. I believe safe containers encourage growth. **Truth Two:** A CrossFit box can be a safe container.

I believe the concepts I have learned as a therapist and life coach can be applied to athletes in helping them with their mental blocks. I believe unlocking one's potential, whether it's in relationships or on the field, is an internal process and not an external one. The purpose of this book is to walk you through that process so you can begin it for yourself.

A sports psychologist teaches imagery, motivation, and attentional focus. I dissect relationships, break thought patterns, and help people rewire cognition. While sports psychologists take more of a scientific approach to the mental game, I take a therapeutic one.

My method as a therapist and life coach is *with* you, not *at* you. I simplify, put things in a shot glass. I push transparency, the unconventional, and shattering false veneers. I build containers, collect stories, and work out of my kitchen. My name is John Kim and I am -

the
angry
therapist

MICRO

Better Performance Techniques.

Inside Out Breathing

We all know the importance of deep breathing. Oxygen in the blood is critical for ATP (Adenosine Triphosphate). ATP is how your body makes energy. To increase oxygen, we must breathe deep from our belly, not our chest. This is called diaphragmatic breathing, which is the only way to get air into the lower third of your lungs. This is where two-thirds of the blood supply is. This breathing technique will increase the efficiency of your lungs. The focus is on inhaling.

Inside Out Breathing is the opposite. You focus in on exhaling.

Swimmers must breathe with precision in order to go fast without swallowing water. Elite swimmers can breathe effortlessly while maintaining perfect form at maximum exertion. Open water swimmers can do the same while fighting waves. Swimmers practice Inside Out Breathing, focusing on a deep exhale instead of a deep inhale.

Each time we take a breath, the air that goes into our lungs is about 21 percent oxygen and only holds a trace of carbon dioxide. The air we exhale is about 14 percent oxygen and nearly 6 percent carbon dioxide. This means when we feel "out of breath", we are not suffering from a lack of oxygen. We only consume about one third of the oxygen we take in. Your body screaming *Stop now!* is actually from an increase in carbon dioxide in your bloodstream.

Focusing on exhaling fully will clear more accumulated carbon dioxide, leaving you feeling like you have more oxygen in your lungs. This process will maintain a sense of relaxation and comfort.

Runner's Block

You've heard of writer's block? Well I suffer from runner's block. I have always been fast, but anything over a mile and I'm gasping for air and cursing my birth. Of course, my technique has a lot to do with it (I tend to run like I'm being chased by the police). But this book is not about technique. One day, out of sheer frustration of getting winded way too fast, I made an exaggerated gasp. A grunt. It was a cry to the Gods. Why can't I run like Jason Bourne?! Every time I ran, I would grunt. This became a habit, an embarrassing one since the people around me would look at me like I had issues.

But then I noticed something. Every time I grunted, I felt a mini reboot. The louder the grunt, the bigger the reboot. A rule of Solution Focused Therapy is to keep doing whatever works without questioning it. So I kept grunting. The more I grunted, the less winded I felt. I was able to keep up my pace and not collapse. Today, my mile is 6:07. Now if I can just run like a sprinter instead of a criminal, I think I can get a sub 6 minute mile.

When I learned about breathing inside out, I realized that by grunting I was focusing on exaggerating my exhale. My "mini reboot" was actually a decrease of carbon dioxide in my bloodstream.

Practice:

1. Start by breathing normally. Exhale by simply releasing rather than actively pushing the air out. You can do both through your nose. Repeat five or six such breaths.

2. Now switch emphasis by actively pushing air out. As you exhale, constrict your throat slightly to produce a rushing sound, loud enough to be heard by someone across the street. Grunt if you have to. As you do, you'll be more conscious of the air passing through your throat than through your nostrils. Repeat 8 to 10 such breaths.

3. Finally, continue your exhale-focused breathing, but consciously shift to making each inhale as passive as possible. See how much of your lungs can you refill simply as a response to the "vacuum" you created with your exhale before needing to switch over to a more active inhale. Repeat until you notice an increase in your ability to refill passively.

As you're doing this, imagine every exhalation as pain leaving your body. The deeper the exhale, the more the pain is released. Literally see the pain, as if it's your breath on a cold Christmas morning.

Experiment with inside out breathing during the warm up run. First, get your heart rate up by jogging. Breathe as you normally do. Then gradually focus on exhaling. Really exaggerate it. Grunt if you have to. Time it with every third step. Notice what happens. Is there a difference? It will feel awkward at first, but push through that.

Once you've trained yourself to breathe this way, apply the technique during a WOD. First, only do it when you're feeling tired and want to stop. Hopefully that's at the end of the WOD and not the beginning. This way, you can see if you're getting a "mini reboot". If that works for you, try to breathe inside out during the entire WOD, from beginning to end. The more you do this, the easier it will become. Don't just do it once and think it's nonsense if you don't feel an instant change. Try it for a week. Do it consistently and pay close attention to the difference.

Process:

Besides what's happening physiologically, breathing inside out allows you to mentally focus on something. When you are running / WODing, focus is key. It takes you out of your thoughts - I'm done! Stop! I can't!- which are generated by false beliefs, based on our story which I will cover in Macro. Therefore, controlled breathing works on two levels, physiologically it keeps you feeling more relaxed and calm and mentally it helps us ignore that screaming voice that causes us to stop.

Visualization (rewire)

"As you think, so shall you become".

- Bruce Lee

There are so many stories out there about the power of visualization. Michael Jordan claims he imagines his shots thousands of times in his head before actually executing them on the court. Skateboarders, gymnast, and snowboarders all visualize their tricks thousands of times, over and over until it happens instinctively. But the question is how much of their success is from visualizing and how much of it is from just plain practice? Is visualization a hokey excuse to cloud science with spirit? Many believe it's just wishful thinking. They believe it's more of a calming exercise than anything. I completely agree that this is possible, but it all depends on execution. If visualization to you means just imagining yourself winning over and over again then yes, it is nothing more than wishful thinking. But if visualization means replaying specific movements under a microscope, mentally examining, tweaking, and reshaping, while anchoring that emotionally, visualization can be an extremely powerful tool. But before we get into techniques of visualization, let's discuss how it works.

When you imagine yourself perfecting your movement and doing what you want with precision, you are in turn physiologically creating neural patterns in your brain, just as if you had physically performed the action. These patterns are similar to small tracks engraved in the brain cells, which can ultimately enable an athlete to perform physical feats by simply mentally practicing the move. This means mental imagery trains our minds and creates the neural patterns in our brain to teach our muscles to do exactly what we want them to do.
During visualization, the brain is directing the target muscles to work in a desired way. This direction creates a neural pattern in the brain, a

pattern identical to the network created by the actual physical performance of the movements. A neural pattern is similar to diagramming the specific wiring and circuits necessary to transmit an electrical current. Alexander Bain (1818–1903) of Great Britain was the first scientist to develop a theory as to how the brain built such patterns to direct and control repeated physical movement. Numerous researchers since that time have expanded on the concept. Visualization alone will not develop the most effective mechanisms in the brain to later perform the desired action, but physical training coupled with visualization will create better recognition of the required nervous system response than physical training alone.

The motor patterns that are generated during imaginary practice are the same as those used for physical practice.

"When confronted with a situation that appears fragmented or impossible, step back, close your eyes, and envision perfection where you saw brokenness. Go to the inner place where there is no problem, and abide in the consciousness of well-being."

- Alan Cohen

I train myself mentally with visualization. The morning of a tournament, before I put my feet on the floor, I visualize myself making perfect runs with emphasis on technique, all the way through to what my personal best is in practice.... The more you work with this type of visualization, especially when you do it on a day-to-day basis, you'll actually begin to feel your muscles contracting at the appropriate times.

- Camille Duvall
(World Professional Slalom Skiing Champion)

Not only can mental imagery improve specific motor skills but it also enhances motivation, mental toughness, and confidence, which will all help elevate your level of execution.

Windmills

I had my first experience with visualization when I was eleven. I was the youngest in a breakdancing crew. I wanted to be as good as the older kids but being the runt of the bunch meant I didn't posses the strength they did. Floor flares were done in my head instead of on cardboard. Any move I couldn't do I would in my head, over and over and over again. I would daydream in classrooms, lie in bed replaying a mental fantasy video of what I couldn't do in real life. A few years later, I would do the same while fantasizing about girls. I wanted to know what it would feel like. During my fantasies, I noticed the placement of my hands, the shift in my body, the whip of my hair. I didn't just see myself doing the moves, I felt it too. Slowly, I was able to execute these moves in real life. Of course it took a lot of practice and they weren't perfect like I had imagined, but what I envisioned came true. I thought it was a gift from God. Maybe it was. But what was also happening was I was making imprints in my brain. I was laying tracks. When I wasn't practicing, I was practicing. I was able to do windmills, hand glides, and buffalo walks. I became a little gymnast without one gymnastic class. Everything was self-taught by observation, visualization, and practice. Today, at 38, I can still do windmills. I do them at weddings and before WODs.

There is no correct way to practice mental imagery. It is all left up to individual preferences and circumstances. But in order for the process to be effective, there must be three factors.

- Relax.

Whether you do it while you're going to bed, standing in the shower half awake, or upside down during your morning meditation, you must be relaxed. Your mind must be clear. Visual imagery requires concentration. If you're tense or your mind is cluttered, the imprint will not be as defined or deep. Paint on a fresh clean canvas.

- Feel it (emotional anchor)

Many visualize the movement but forget to attach an emotional element. They see it but don't feel it. They are focused on the product (time / score) rather than the experience. This process is not as effective. Think about the difference between a powerful dream and a movie. Films may move you, but you usually snap back into reality as you're leaving the theater. A powerful dream can stay with you for days or even weeks. It lingers. The reason is when we're dreaming, we are not just watching, we are experiencing. How many times have you woken up with a crush on someone you didn't care for before the dream? Feelings leave impressions. So feel the air, your breath, and your heart. Notice the clock, the people around you. Take in the smell, the sounds, the energy in the room. But most importantly, feel what's coming up for you while you are doing the movement. Not what you're thinking but what you are feeling. If you're feeling ambivalence, unsure, insecure, think of a time when you felt completely certain and unstoppable. While you're visualizing, replace your negative feelings with the positive. Notice the old exiting your body as you fill up with the new. Feel the power, in your feet, legs, stomach, shoulders, arm, grip, and mind. Remember this feeling. You will bring it up like a skilled actor when you're executing the exercise in the box. Remember, the richer the experience, the deeper the imprint.

- Focus on Details

Put your execution under a microscope. Notice the mistakes in your form, your grip, your stance. Examine it. See the mistake. Closer. Notice what that feels like when you play it. Stop. Pause. Rewind. Replay, but now fix it. See the fix. Feel the difference. Notice the inch adjustment in your foot position, the slight turn of your neck, the straightening of your posture. Get precise like you're a watch maker fixing a watch. Focus on every aspect of the move, every single detail, from head to toe. The more specific the intention, the more specific the results. Remember whatever you believe is what your body will do. So when you are thinking of your intention make sure it is clear, specific, and achievable.

Practice:

The Spotlight of Excellence

Imagine a huge spotlight beaming down on the floor one meter in front of you. The light beam is about a meter in diameter. Now think back to a time when you were performing at the very peak of your ability. Each movement you made brought about a successful outcome and everything just seemed to flow without much conscious effort. You are in a dissociated state. You are looking at yourself from the outside. Examine each of your five senses. See yourself inside the circle and excelling. Imagine exactly what the 'you' inside the circle is seeing, hearing, feeling, and smelling. Notice the 'taste of success' in your mouth.

Now step into the spotlight and become fully associated so that you are experiencing events through your own eyes and in real time. Again, notice what you are seeing, hearing, feeling, smelling and tasting. Notice exactly what this feels like so that you can reproduce it at will whenever your confidence is waning.

While you're lying in bed, after you've check your box's WOD for the next day, run through the entire WOD in your head. We both know you do this anyway. Use the visualization techniques mentioned above. Replay every single movement. Go through it thoroughly. If the WOD involves an exercise you are not good at, put it under a microscope, fix the mistakes in your head, notice, feel, experience the change. See the carbon dioxide leaving your body as you breath inside out. See yourself doing it at a record-breaking time. Do this every single night. Make it a routine. Know that you are not just fantasizing, but actually laying tracks.

Your performance may never line up perfectly with what you envision but that's not the goal. The goal is to use mental imagery as a dangling carrot, to chase something, to keep improving.

Imagery to Fight Fear

Sometimes we have to do a lift or exercise that we are not good at. For me, it's anything overhead. For some, it may be a front squat, a muscle up, or box jump that left a scar down your shin once. Chances are, fear will stand in the way of your execution, especially when you are tired. For example, you may be doing okay with front squats until the third round when you begin to lean forward and drop the bar before you can finish a rep. So you step back and take a breath. Within this split second, fear oozes in like a poisonous gas. Now as you approach the bar, you are not only tired, you are afraid. This fear causes you to drop the bar again. This is an external (temporary) mental block and it will get worse and worse unless you address it.

This is when imagery can be helpful. The second you notice fear creeping in, step back and imagine yourself doing it. Play it back fast. The clock is running. See it in your head. Turn that image into a belief as if you're just replaying what you've already done. Before fear gets it's grip on you, step back in and do it again. When you're doing it, use what you've just imagined as a blueprint that you are now just tracing. The more you use imagery to fight fear, the less power fear will have over you while you are at your weakest.

Process:

The brain is divided into two sides. The left is the logical side (words, logic, rational thought). The right is the creative side (imagination and intuition). Most of the day, we are using our left, logical side. Day to day tasks, bills, work, etc. By exercising the right side, the creative side of the brain, we actually restore balance in the brain. This allows access to the mind-body connection to achieve what you want. Visualization targets the right side of your brain, so mental imagery strengthens the mind-body connection.

Mind power is the second greatest power next to the spirit. Thoughts can manifest physically. For example, negative thoughts and emotions lower the immune system, while positive thought and emotions actually boost the immune system. When you visualize, you are creating positive thought.

Visualization makes neural patterns in your brain, restores balance to achieve a better mind-body connection, and creates a conduit to funnel positive thought.

The Power of Numbers

CrossFit is a numbers game. Times, reps, weight, rounds, and numbers can be intimidating. Behind intimidation is fear. Fear creates mental blocks. Actually, mental blocks stem from false beliefs and false beliefs is what generates the fear. But we'll get into that later. Right now, let's just stick with fear.

Which work out looks more difficult?

A) 100 pull ups, 150 push ups, 200 sit ups, and 250 squats.

Or

B) 20 pull ups, 30 push ups, 40 sit ups, 50 squats for 5 rounds.

Most people would say A. Many see 100 pull ups and wonder if that's possible for them. And, if so, how long that would even take. Mentally, there's already a block. A "I can't" flag has just been tossed into the air. Even if it doesn't stop you, that mental stutter step can affect your performance. This happens every day in CrossFit. We all see a workout that intimidates us. This allows space for discouragement and doubt. One way to minimize that stutter step and help you push through during the workout is to focus on number sets.

Although workout A and B have the exact same number of reps per exercise, seeing workout B broken into pieces, in this case rounds, tells our brain it's easier even if logically we know it's not. Your internal dialogue may go something like this: "I know I can do 20 pull ups. So I just have to break it up into four sets of 5. And I've done

10 unbroken push ups before. I just have to do 3 sets of them. When we break things into pieces, mountains become hills. Changing the size of the mountain will trick your brain and encourage you to run toward instead of away.

My Greatest Chipper

In order to be licensed as a Marriage Family Therapist, one must receive a Masters in Psychology, log in 3000 face to face therapy hours (family, group, individual) / supervision, then take two exams. One is 4 hours long with 200 questions and the other is 2 hours long with 40 questions.

I looked at this and instantly thought it was a mountain I could not climb. I've been a C student most of my life and vowed to never go back to school after college. Red flags were thrown up left and right. "I can't. There's no way. I'm not smart enough." It would also be my third career so the amount of time it would take to achieve this would also be a factor. My brain was screaming "no!".

The way I got through it was by using the power of numbers.

I knew I could take 12 units, especially if they were classes I was genuinely passionate about. Could I do it 4 times? Maybe. What about providing 3000 hours of therapy? That seemed like a lifetime. But if you break it down, it's about 5 hours of therapy a day. This seemed manageable. Could I do it for 2 and a half years? Only if I got paid for it. That would mean I would need to work at a treatment center as a Marriage Family Therapist Intern for about 2 and a half years. Okay. What's next? Just two exams. That doesn't sound bad. But for someone who was called down to the principal's office to discuss his shockingly poor SAT scores, it would be a giant wall. The fact that it's a four hour exam is what intimidates me. But I knew that if I could mentally break it down into four one hour exams, I might be able to get through it. And if I could get through that, then I can surely take a two hour exam.

My chipper was broken down into taking 12 units of classes I was passionate about 4 times. Then working at a treatment center for about 2 1/2 years. And finally, taking two exams. I'm not going to lie. It was painstakingly difficult, I got distracted somewhere in the middle, and it took me nearly 6 years. But I got through it. Today, I am licensed.

Everyone has a chipper story. Not just me. Breaking down an overwhelming task into manageable pieces is a concept that dates back to the pyramids. But the way it's broken down is different for each individual. It depends on what number sets will encourage traction.

Here's what works for me:

If there's a workout with the number 50, I ignore the 50 and just focus on getting to 30. I literally convince myself I just need to do 30. After I hit 30, I tell myself I can do 10 more as if it's extra credit. Then the final 10 is a countdown in my head. I tell myself I can stop after 10 seconds. This numbers set is helpful when it's an exercise I struggle with, like wall balls.

At 5'7, I don't have the reach that many others do. This means I'd rather swallow needles than row. Rowing feels never ending to me, like I'm on a treadmill. Therefore, I translate meters into pulls. By changing the unit of measurement, it exercise becomes more manageable. I don't see distance, but I do see pulls. Now I apply a number set. For example, if I have to row 1000m, I just say I have to pull 25 times for 4 sets because I know that 25 pulls is approximately 250 meters. Even if it takes me more than 25 pulls, which it usually does, I stay with that number so I don't let myself slide.

Now I do my number set with the wall balls, ignore the 50 and just focus on 30. I do 30 hard pulls. Once I get to 30, 10 more for extra credit, then a 10 second count down. I do that process 4 times and I've rowed 1000 meters. Of course, I may fall short and have to do some extra pulls. But at that point I'm so close to finishing, it's just a sprint to the line.

Practice:

Come up with your own number set. For many, it's sets of 10s. They break everything up into 10 reps. But you will have different sets for different workouts. My number set for Fran (21-15-9 thrusters / pull ups) is different than Karen (150 wall balls). For Fran, I know I can do the first 21 reps of thrusters / pull ups unbroken. It's the 15 that I struggle with. So my number set doesn't even kick in until I've started the 15. My number set is 10. I just focus on getting to 10. Nothing else. For Karen, my number set begins right away. I just focus on getting 30 wall balls unbroken. Then 10. Then I begin my 10 second count down. Once I've done 50, my number set becomes 10. I just focus on getting 10 unbroken wall balls before I allow myself to rest. I may not get to 10 but that's where I set my numbers. I do this until the workout is over. As I get better with wall balls, I will change my number set to 15 or 20 after I finish the first 50. I call this tightening the vice.

Figure out what works for you. Create your own number set for every WOD. Experiment with the sets. Then slowly tighten the vice.

As you stand in front of the whiteboard reviewing the WOD you've already replayed in your head a thousand times the night before while doing your mental imagery work, lock in your number set.

Reframe the reps and structure it so it caters to your strengths.

Bleed Number Sets

Many stop at the end of a set. For example, in a 21-15-9 workout, one may stop after her last rep of 21. Then after 15. And after 9. Those would be the obvious times to take a quick break. Our brain automatically tells us we've accomplished a set. Now you deserve a rest. Or say you're doing a WOD where there are 10 reps of something, then 9, then 8, etc.. We usually stop after we finish each number, even if it's just for a second. Bleeding means to continue onto the next number set before stopping. So after finishing 10, you would move on to the set of 9 without any rest. You may only get one or two more reps in, but that's okay. The key is to train your brain to not stop in between the number sets. If we stop after a number set, our sense of accomplishment allows our body to rest longer. We get comfortable really fast. If we stop in the middle of a number set, 21 or 15 or 10, we don't allow ourselves to rest as much. This is because in our mind, we are not finished. We know we are the middle of something. The set is not complete.

After the WOD, ask yourself if it was helpful. Did your number set provide traction? Did focusing on hitting your marks get you out of your

thoughts? Were you able to go longer? Faster?
Was your number set too easy? Too difficult?

Continue this process. Do it for every WOD.
You'll get a feel for what sets work and don't
work. Remember, it's not just about getting a
better time or more reps. You are sharpening
your ability to focus as well as strengthening
mental muscles to stay out of your head.
Strengthening your "out of your head" muscles
will benefit you not only in the box but also out.
We will discuss more of this in Macro.

Process:

By using number sets, you are doing two things.
One, you are reframing. Two, you are getting
out of your thoughts. Reframing is a technique
used in psychotherapy to help clients see their
situation in a new light, from a different
perspective. Wearing this new lens can create a
boost of mental strength. Reframing the reps
and rounds in your mind by focusing on a
specifically designed set that appears more
achievable encourages desired behavior. The
screaming "I can't" voice head turns into "I can
probably", which leads me to the second piece,
getting out of your head. Most heads are filled
with negative thoughts. This is due to your
perception of yourself. Your beliefs are formed
from your story and no one has a perfect story.
Therefore, your mind is clustered with distorted,
false, and negative thoughts. When there is

challenge and conflict is when these thoughts are the loudest. In this case, the challenge is a physical one and our negative thoughts come charging at us, preventing us from our potential. Focusing on your count and hitting that number pulls you out of your head, which prevents you from having those thoughts. Basically, you're distracting your self. But you are also training your mind to focus and be in the present. The more you are able to do this, the more mental strength you will have to push through when you would usually quit.

Stretch Your White Zone

I tell my clients growth happens in that space where you are able to get comfortable with the uncomfortable. In my world, uncomfortable may mean examining one's defects, communication style, being vulnerable, exploring their addiction to validation, etc. Most don't like being in this space let alone trying to get comfortable there, which is why most people don't grow.

I believe the same concept can be applied to CrossFit, especially metcons. Growth happens when you are able to take what is uncomfortable and make it comfortable, or more comfortable. The more you are able to do this, the faster you will be. Someone who is comfortable with discomfort will go much further than someone who is not. At the end of discomfort is what

CrossFiters call a wall. We all have walls. Some just have pushed their wall much further.

I call the space just as you are hitting your wall the white zone. It's when you're exhausted and don't think you can go any longer. It usually comes in the last 30 seconds of the WOD or, for some, during the warm up. When you enter this zone, try to stay in it as long as you can. Stretch it. Make that the challenge. Know that stretching this is what will make you stronger and faster.

Practice:

While you're doing your warm up run, get to your white zone as fast as you can. You may explode out of the gates like a muzzled greyhound and people may think you're an idiot for trying to race during the warm up. Or at least that's what happens to me. Hopefully, you will also be grunting (breathing inside out).

I suggest first exercising your white zone during a warm up run so that you have the luxury to slow down or go faster. You can experiment with that space without fully exerting yourself.

Once you've gotten to your white zone, notice what you are thinking, feeling, the broken record playing in your head. Remember this. Mark it. Now, during a WOD, notice when you reach that marker. You will know if you've marked it. Then once you reach it, do everything you can to stretch it. This means stay in the white zone as long as you possibly can.

Continue this process over and over, each time trying to stretch that space. The more you can stretch your white zone, get comfortable with being uncomfortable, the faster you will be.

Process:

On the surface you are focusing on a task but what's happening underneath is you are mentally distracting yourself. Using a visual measurement (white zone) allows you to get out of your head, the thoughts and voices that order your body to stop. You've heard this statement a million times: Your body can go much longer than you think it can. This is another way of tricking your body to do so.

Most people are afraid of getting to that tired place. They resist it. Things are fun until it gets difficult. Stretching your white zone changes that mindset. In encourages you to play in that space. The more you play / stretch that space, the less fear you will have of it. Remember, fear is a mental block. Many stop because they are scared.

Trigger Words

We discussed the power of numbers. Now let's talk about the power of words. Actually, the power of emotions. The word will only act as a trigger.

We've all heard of stories of extraordinary human strength. The mother lifting a tree off her son's leg. Ship wrecked survivors enduring the ocean for a week. A trapped rock climber cutting off his own arm to escape.

This strength is released by an adrenaline rush, the fight or flight response of the adrenal gland. This response is our body's primitive, automatic, inborn response that prepares the body to "fight" or "flee" from perceived attack, harm or threat to our survival. In this state, the adrenal glad releases adrenaline (epinephrine). This process releases dopamine, a natural pain killer. An adrenaline rush causes the muscles to perform respiration at an increased rate improving strength. Nerve cells fire, chemicals are released, and our body undergoes a series of changes. Our respiratory rate increases. Blood is shunted away from our digestive tract and directed into our muscles and limbs, giving us extra energy. Our pupils dilate. Our awareness intensifies. Our sight sharpens. Our impulses quicken. Our perception of pain diminishes. Our immune system mobilizes with increased activation. We become prepared—physically and psychologically—for fight or flight.

I believe we can tap into this fight or flight state without being physically in danger or threatened. There is another door. It's labeled "I'm mad at you," or our emotional state. Emotions can be extremely powerful. They can have the same "fight or flight" effect on our body. They can release an adrenaline rush.

A Broken Shower

When I was fourteen, we lived in a house where the bathroom light switch was on the outside of the bathroom. No, this was not in Korea. I have no idea who thought of placing it there, but it contributed to my parents rushing me to the hospital to get stitches in my foot one night. While I was in the shower, my brother thought it would be funny to flick the light on and off. The more he did it, the more furious I became. I don't remember, but I guess I kicked the shower door because it shattered like Bruce Lee was standing behind it. No, I don't know karate and there was no pain. The glass door felt as if it was made of Balsa wood. Of course, later it would hurt. A lot. But at the time, dopamine was my shield and the adrenaline rush released by my anger (emotion) was my sword.

How many times have you punched something because you were angry with your boyfriend, then surprised at the damage on the wall? How many times have you WODed longer, faster, harder because you were thinking about your ex's cheating face, the soccer coach that didn't believing in you, or the kid that bullied you all through junior high. Using your recent break up to go ape shit during a WOD can be cathartic and the adrenaline released from your emotional state can be powerful. But it can also be dangerous. Instead of processing your emotion, you are stirring, bringing up, and this can create residue, which can ultimately be a giant mental block.

Anger is the easiest way to get your shot glass of adrenaline. But the consequences outweigh the rewards. You are risking what comes up during the workout to leak into other areas of your life. This is what I mean by residue. It is surfacing because it is not resolved. This energy is negative. It will make you moody and affect the relationships around you, not only in the box but at home, work, etc. Are you willing to lower your quality of life for a better time?

There is a way to receive that adrenaline rush from a positive source. For many, including myself, CrossFit has been a bookmark in our lives. This new lifestyle has separated the old from the new. It has closed an old chapter and opened a new one, sparked a rebirth. CrossFit has given us a new lens to see ourselves through.

Review your story and notice the old you (before CrossFit) and the new you (after CrossFit).

What is it about the new you that you like? Instead of anger or resentment, focus on this new version of yourself and how valuable that is to you. Think about how much work you've put in, how much shit you've had to go through to get here. Would you let someone take it away? I don't know about you, but my answer is over my dead body. This is the mindset during each WOD. This is what's at stake. It's not anger or resentment. It's determination. It's a non-negotiating stance to lean forward. It's knowing what you've built up until this point and not being willing to let that go. This is the emotional keg that must be tapped.

Practice:

What words trigger not wanting to go back to the old you? One way to think about this is to ask yourself what words remind you of the old you? Out of those words, which one tugs at you the most on an emotional level? Remember, this is not about others. It's about you and your journey. No one else's.

Here are a few examples of trigger words.

- Not afraid anymore.

- Never again.

- Not going back.

- Climb.

- Grow.

- Rebirth.

Decide what word or phrase works for you. Everyone's will be different, depending on our story. Once you have chosen your words or phrases, drop them in front of you during the WOD like they're iron curtains. See the old you as if you were watching a movie. Imagine that point in your life when you had the most fear, felt you were the weakest, when you didn't like yourself. It might have been ten years ago when you were in that dysfunctional relationship or just yesterday alone in your room.

Know that the harder you push, the more distance you will have from that version of you. There needs to be an emotional connection so it's not just about seeing it. You must feel it. Underneath this feeling is a river of adrenaline. Use it. It's yours.

Climb.

Grow.

Rebirth.

You can also use this technique before the WOD to warm up your mental and emotional engine, be filled with 92 octane of determination, and to put that adrenaline on reserve for what's to come. It can be a quick meditation exercise without looking like you're meditating. Start the internal dialogue while you're staring at the WOD or rolling out. But make sure you do it after you've socialized so that you are focused and not distracted.

Process:

When I'm giving therapy, sometimes I split the client identity into two, the old and the new. I make sure there is a distinct divide between what was and what is. It is helpful for the client to see this separation. This mindset encourages one to work toward something new rather than dwell on the old. There is pain in everyone's past no matter how "perfect" their life is. I use that pain and emotion as leverage to rewrite their story. The harder they work, the stronger their resistance to going back to their old story, dysfunctional behavior, and false beliefs about themselves (who they were). I call this process emotional leveraging and I believe it can be used as a tool to enhance performance for athletes without the danger of building emotional residue.

See / Save Energy

Imagine that you hold a source of super power energy in your core, somewhere in your abdomen or hip area. Color it so it's bright so that you can see it. This energy is not unlimited. Like gasoline in your car, it runs out during each WOD. Imagine that every every time you break form, compromise technique, look up, this energy leaks out of your body. So the goal is to keep this energy inside. Trap it and DO NOT let it leak. See it distribute through out your body when you need it. See it shoot from your hips to your palms in a split second when you do a thruster, from your knees to your triceps during a muscle up, contained solid when you're running with perform form. Focus on this energy. Notice it. Feel it. See it. Use it.

PROCESS

Visualizing your energy can be a powerful tool. It syncs mind with body. This process keeps you focused on form and allows you to get the maximum results with explosive movements.

Now that you've had your sweets, it's time to eat your protein.

MACRO

What are mental blocks?

I define a mental block as any thought or feeling that prevents us from our desired behavior and potential. It doesn't matter if we're referring to relationships or doing our max number of butterfly pull-ups.

There are two types of mental blocks.

External Mental Blocks

External mental blocks are temporary thoughts and feelings we bring into the box. They may arise from getting into an argument with the guy that just cut you off or a stressful day at work. You may be experiencing PMS or an expiring marriage. External mental blocks may stem from relationships but not the relationship you have with yourself. External mental blocks are not ingrained. They are outside of self. They are temporary. They come and go. Therefore, they will not be my focus.

Internal Mental Blocks

Internal mental blocks are thoughts and feelings that arise from our core. They are ingrained. They were created from our story - upbringing, relationships (abuse), random events (trauma), failures and accomplishments, break ups. Depending on our tools, the way we cope with these events and relationships is through our addiction or addictive behavior, drugs, sex, love, food, gambling, cutting, and of course, exercise.

We may not all be addicts but we all have vices. Some struggle with them more than others. We also all have false beliefs about ourselves. It doesn't matter if you're going to the CrossFit Games or just getting your first double under. Everyone has some form or pattern of distorted cognitions because no one has a "perfect" story. Our story forms a distinctive lens we see the world through and, more importantly, how we view ourselves. We don't see the world as it is. We see the world as we are. So mental blocks are about dirty lenses. In order to rid ourselves of these blocks, we must clean our lenses. We must dissolve these false beliefs about ourselves.

Someone once asked me, "How do we know the beliefs are false if we believe them?"

We all have a Pseudo and Solid Self, a term created by Marty Bowen in regards to family dynamics and differentiation of self. To Bowen, the degree to which a differentiation of self occurs in an individual reflects the extent to which that person is able to distinguish between the intellectual process and the feeling process (emotions) he or she is experiencing. Thus differentiation of self is related to the degree to which one is able to choose between having his or her actions, relationships and life guided by feelings or thoughts (What part of me is running my life – my gut or my brain? Who is in charge - my feelings or my thinking?)

I define Pseudo as false and Solid as truth. When you are maneuvering in Pseudo Self, you may be seeking approval and validation. Pseudo is fed by ego. Solid is transparency. Pseudo wants you to live in your head while Solid Self wants you to live in the present. Pseudo wants you to negotiate or question yourself. Solid wants you to accept and live your truth. Everyone struggles with this inner conflict. In the box, your Pseudo Self is obsessed with the Leaderboard. It forces you to compare yourself to others. It constantly seeks approval and validation. It digs up your past and throws it in your face. It creates false beliefs. *I'm not good enough. Fast enough. Strong enough. I can't. I don't deserve it.* Our Solid Self accepts and encourages. *I can. I will. I don't care what others think.* It's our Solid Self that tells us that a belief is false.

What if you don't have a Solid Self? Everyone has a Solid Self. We are not born with cognitive

distortions. Life creates them for us. Your Solid Self may not be loud but it's there. You just have to listen for it. We don't usually hear it because we're not used to listening to it. Listening to it means challenging our thoughts.
The goal is strengthen your Solid Self and cripple your Pseudo Self. By doing this, you will gradually be rid of your false beliefs. Doing away with your false beliefs dissolves your mental blocks. By dissolving your mental blocks, you will perform in a truer form. By performing in your truest form, you will have the most potential.

When you are in your truest form is when you have the most potential. **Truth Three**. I believe this for every aspect of your life, including your athletic abilities.

So how does one get in their truest form?

First, what are your false beliefs?

Here are a few of mine.

- *Since I didn't play sports in high school or college, I am not an athlete.*

- *I am too small to compete in CrossFit.*

- *Being a Marriage Family Therapist and not a sports psychologist disqualifies me to write about this topic.*

What are yours?

Note: It is important to actually write this out instead of just thinking about them. The hood is open and we are exploring your engine. In order to fix it or make it go faster, we must know what the problem is, what is blocking it from maximum out-put. Write it down.

_____

_____

_____

_____

_____

_____

_____

_____

_____

_____

Where do these beliefs stem from?

- Since I didn't play sports in high school or college, I am not an athlete.

Technically, I was on the high school football team but I wasn't *really* on the team. I was on special teams and I only made one tackle the entire two years of my football career. It was a famous tackle titled "The Korean Finger Tackle" by the coach himself and became the butt of jokes in the locker room. A horrible sports experience in high school formed my false belief.

- I am too small to compete in CrossFit.

I've always been the little guy. Because of my size, I wasn't the first one picked when it came to sports. I tried to make up for it by focusing on speed instead of strength. This mental block kept me away from squats, dead lifts, and presses - the weight room. Instead, I concentrated on sports that require balance and agility, like breakdancing, skateboarding, and snowboarding. This kept me from getting stronger.

Today I am 38 years old. I am done growing physically. I am 5'7 and a buck fifty. These are facts. They are not in my head. But what is in my head is the belief that because of my size, I can't "play". I can CrossFit but I'll never be able to complete. This ingrained belief is based on my story and how I viewed myself in comparison to "real" athletes.

- Being a marriage family therapist instead of a sports psychologist disqualifies me to write about this topic.

People in my field don't focus on helping their clients get faster WOD times. We work with reducing anxiety from expired relationships and family conflict. We work with addicts in recovery. This label creates a false belief that I am not qualified. My theories are invalid. My false belief stems from my view on what society defines as qualified.

Where do you believe your false beliefs stem from? Write it down. Don't worry. No one will see this except you.

_____

_____

_____

_____

_____

_____

_____

How do these false beliefs manifest in your thoughts and behavior today?

- Since I didn't play sports in high school or college, I am not an athlete.

Today I am surrounded by the guys who scored touchdowns, won state championships, and became heroes, while I watched from the sideline. Although I can keep up with many of them in the box, there is a distinct separation in my mind between them and me due to our athletic resume. I still see myself on special teams.

This false belief defines me as less than. It puts me on a mental bench. I feel like I don't belong. It's cause me to compare my self to "real" athletes and prevents me from giving it my all. These thoughts and feelings manifests in slower times, lifting less weight, etc.

- I am too small to compete in CrossFit.

This false belief prevents me from going into heavy lifting WODs with confidence. I disqualify myself and line my performance with fear. This fear prevents me from getting stronger and competing. Basically, it keeps me trapped inside a bubble. There is a limit to how far I believe I can go in CrossFit. *I can do it for fun. But that's it.*

- Being a marriage family therapist instead of a sports psychologist disqualifies me to write about this topic.

This false belief makes me question myself. It tells me no one will read this and, if they do, it will not help them. It makes me feel like a fraud. These thoughts discourage me, making it extremely difficult to get up each morning and work on this book. My false belief makes it hard to write this book.

How do your false beliefs manifest in your thoughts and behavior today?

_____

_____

_____

_____

_____

_____

_____

_____

Now Reframe.

Every false belief you wrote down came from your Pseudo Self. They are distorted truths and false perceptions based on your story. It's this constant inner conflict between your Pseudo and Solid Self that creates mental hiccups, speed bumps, and blocks.

Try reframing your false beliefs by pulling from your Solid Self. If it helps, imagine that you are someone else, like a best friend, so your reasoning won't be slanted by your self-perception. For some, it's much easier to look in from another person's perspective. For example, being able to compliment others but not themselves.

Here are my reframes.

- *Since I didn't play sports in high school or college, I am not an athlete.*

The fact that I didn't play many sports in high school or college doesn't mean I am not an athlete today. It just means I didn't play many sports in high school or college. What makes me an athlete today isn't based on my history but rather my current involvement in athletics.

- *I am too small to compete in CrossFit.*

Two words. Chris Spealler.

- Being a marriage family therapist instead of a sports psychologist disqualifies me to write about this topic.

Being a marriage family therapist instead of a sports psychologist gives this topic a fresh new angle. It may help some or it may not, but it's my take and my truth. I believe in what I am writing. That is my qualification, not the letters after my name.

Reframe your false beliefs.

_____

_____

_____

_____

_____

_____

_____

_____

_____

How did you feel when you reframed it? What came up for you?

For me, it felt good to say it out loud and write it down. This process allowed me to see the difference in my thoughts and thinking. However, just because I say or write something doesn't mean I believe it.

I will save trees and assume you felt the same.

Knowing where your false belief came from is only half the coin. The other half is asking yourself how you felt when that happened and how that feeling is associated to what's happening in the box now. This is called processing. Or, simply put, therapy.

So go back and really notice what comes up for you when you explore where your false beliefs came from.

Let's go back to my example. When I think about being on that bench in high school, I remember that it made me feel inadequate, less than, weak, inferior, and powerless. Looking back at it now, I kind of feel sorry for myself. I see this little guy without a single mark on his uniform and it makes me sad. I wish I could go back and be better.

In the box, when I compare myself to all the athletes, these same feelings begin to come up.

Weak, less than, inferior, and powerless. The same thing happens when we visit our parents. We snap back into that rebellious thirteen-year old, or the quiet kid that wasn't able to express herself.

I compete with the athletes because I don't want to feel weak and powerless. But this competitive mindset is not coming from a healthy place. I have attached meaning. It's loaded. Because of my false belief, this WOD means.

If I beat them, I'm no longer a bench warmer.

That's the connection. This is the problem, the faulty wiring. This is the false belief that will set me up for a huge fall.

If I win, I will only reinforce the sentence above. I will put added pressure to keep winning every WOD. One day, I will not "win". But instead of it being just another WOD, it means I am a bench warmer. Then I will internalize this, be disappointed in myself, and create more false beliefs while re-enforcing others. I am not good enough. I am not strong enough. I am NOT an athlete.

In order to stop this cycle of thinking, there needs to be a form of closure. In relationships, we must accept and forgive so that we can move on without bringing anger and pain from our previous relationship into the new one. The same thing needs to happen here. What would acceptance and forgiveness look like for you?

For me, it would mean going back to that kid in high school and telling him that not being first string on the football team doesn't make you powerless or weak. It would mean to tell myself today that I am not that kid in high school and I don't have to prove myself to anyone. It would mean telling myself I am an athlete because I go into the box every day and give it my all. Not because I get a faster time than someone.

Of course, me saying this to myself isn't going to change my thinking or perspective and dissolve my mental blocks overnight. But it will begin the process, and that's what's important. Like I said in the beginning, dissolving mental blocks is a process. My goal in writing this book is to be a catalyst, spark revelations, to connect dots, to begin the process of closure - acceptance and forgiveness.

Maneuver in your Solid Self. What does that look like in the box?

For me, it means no more comparing myself to others. It means being okay with my score. It means working on my weakness. It means knowing when to push and when to stop. It means constantly reminding myself that my performance doesn't define me. It means giving instead of taking, which I will discuss later.

Now execute it.

I try daily.

The more you invest in this process, the more strength you will have to maneuver in Solid Self. This process will rid your mental blocks, creating better performance and, more importantly, a better experience.

In Action

There's a girl I know. Let's call her Stacey. Whenever I tried to encourage her during a WOD, instead of pushing herself harder she would get angry and slow down. I talked to her about this. During our conversation we realized what was happening. As a kid, she never received praise. She only got "you're not good enough". So when I was trying to push her, she was not hearing encouragement. She was hearing what she was conditioned to hearing, "You're not doing it right. You're not good enough". The attention made her shrink. She couldn't hear encouragement as encouragement. She heard it as criticism. This mental block, which stems from a false belief that she is not good enough, hindered her performance. Me pushing her was the trigger that released this false belief.

Once we realized where this was coming from, we were able to connect the dots. She was able to see how her false beliefs, based on her story and relationship with her parents, affected her performance in the box. Now that she was able to detect the false belief, she had to reframe. Her worth has nothing to do with her ability or performance. This began the process of acceptance ans forgiveness. For her, it was accepting and forgiving not only her parents, but also herself. The more she was able to do this, the better her performance got in the box.

"Tell me what you fear and I will tell you what has happened to you."

- D.W. Winnicott

Review

STEP ONE

What are your false beliefs?

- If I'm not the best, it's not even worth doing.
- This is a boy's game.
- If I don't crush WODS, I am not an athlete.
- Since I am a coach, I have to be better than the members.
- I'm not strong enough.
- I'm not fast enough.
- I'm too tall.
- I'm too short.

- I'm too old.
- If I don't RX, I have failed.
- If I don't win, I'm nothing.
- I don't deserve to be good at something.
- I can't.

STEP TWO

Where do these beliefs stem from?

We are not born with false beliefs. They accumulate through our story. Dig. Find the source. Replay your life and discover when you first had that belief. What was the event that formed it? Maybe it was what someone said or how they treated you?

STEP THREE

How do these false beliefs manifest in your thoughts and behavior?

Avoidance? Burying yourself? Short temper? Burn out? Injury? Self-destructive behavior? Shutting down? Withdrawing? Comparing? Seeking approval or validation? There are patterns. Find them. Chances are, they are not only happening during CrossFit. They occur or have been occurring in other areas of your life.

STEP FOUR

Reframe.

Pull from your Solid Self. How would your Solid Self rephrase it? Flip the script.

STEP FIVE

Now attach emotion. How do you feel when you think about where your false belief came from? What meaning did you attach to it? What comes up for you when you think about that? How you do carry that with you today? How does it impact you emotionally today? Do you feel about yourself because of this?

STEP SIX

Rewire

Accept and forgive. What ever that looks like for you. Know that it's a process. It doesn't happen over night.

STEP SEVEN

Maneuver in your Solid Self. What does that look like in the box?

STEP EIGHT

Execute it. One day at a time.

Of course it would help if you executed this process with a therapist, but you don't have to.

You can do a lot of this on your own. Just make sure you write it down. Thinking about it isn't enough. You have to be honest with yourself or you're wasting your time. Think of it as an emotional WOD. The more you do it, the more revelations you will have. With these revelations, you will be able to notice unhealthy thought patterns and cognitive distortions. You will be able to break them, changing the behavior.

Whether you do it alone, with a therapist, or other CrossFitters, what you are doing is rewiring. You are taking apart years and years of unhealthy thinking and putting it back together in a new way so that you can run smoother. This is not easy, nor is it fast. It will be painful. But, where is there growth without pain?

The good news is the mental and emotional work you do on yourself bleeds into all areas of your life. Although your motivation for change may be better performance in CrossFit, the results will directly affect all of your relationships. Most importantly, the one you have with yourself.

Now back to the question, *how do you get into your truest form?* You don't "get" into your truest form. There is no button. There is only a process. But it is impossible to be in your truest form at all times. It's like perfection. We can only strive for it. **Truth Four.**

Common Archetypes

These are some common archetypes I have seen in the box. Can you relate to any?

The Ex-Athlete

You were a track star in high school. Or a first string quarterback in college, state champion wrestler, gymnast, rower, etc. You've been praised for your athletic ability most of your life. But for whatever reason, you didn't make it "to the top" or professional level. Maybe you didn't want it. Maybe you weren't good enough. Maybe you started to define your worth by your ability and "walking off the field" was a choice toward growth. Then you find CrossFit and suddenly it all comes back. Praise, high fives, recognition, and worth. It's an amazing feeling. You forget how much you missed it.

Now you're putting pressure on yourself. People expect high scores because you're killing everything. This feeds into your ego, or your Pseudo Self, and false beliefs begin to form. Many even smell familiar. Once again, your worth is contingent on your ability and performance. Another false belief may be that this is your last chance to be "on top" and you're not going to fuck it up this time! You are now going into the box loaded. Every single WOD is a make or break instead of a progression. This mindset might be a turbo for you. But it is a dangerous place to be. If you don't meet your or others' expectations, or if someone knocks you off the board, that drop is a long and hard one. Then you internalize, which only builds more pressure inside your mental crock-pot. You go into WODs with anger, fear, and negative energy. You may not realize, but people can feel it. It's like a virus. It starts infecting some of the relationships you have inside and outside the box. The more you continue this cycle, the bigger the mental blocks become until one day you wake up and realize it's not worth it. You don't enjoy it anymore. You've come full circle. This is why you hung up your jersey the first time.

What are your false beliefs? Where do they stem from (the source)? How do your false beliefs manifest in your thoughts or behavior?

Reframe

The truth is that you have an edge because of your athletic ability and history. This is a gift, not a curse, depending on your perspective. Instead of your history having power over you, CrossFit can be the catalyst that finally takes that power back. Again, a gift. This is what's at stake. It's not just about being number one. Maybe you can finally enjoy a sport by finding nectar in the process instead of the product. Remember, change is about breaking patterns. This is your opportunity to break this pattern and grow.

Now attach emotion. How do you feel when you think about where your false belief came from? What meaning did you attach to it? What comes up for you when you think about that? How do you carry that with you today? How does it impact you emotionally? How do you feel about yourself because of this?

Rewire.

Accept. Accept your false beliefs and how they have been infecting your thoughts, behavior, relationships, performance, and happiness – your quality of life.

Forgive. Forgive your coach, your parents, your boyfriend, yourself. Know what was your piece and what was theirs. Maybe the pressures they put on you had to do with what they wanted, not what you wanted. Maybe they were trying to make up for something they were lacking in their life. Know that you are starting a new chapter now with CrossFit and this time you will maneuver in your Solid Self. What does that look like for you?

- Not comparing my self or my story with others?
- Not pushing myself to injury?
- Not having to prove anything?
- Focusing on having fun?

- Knowing that fun doesn't mean not training, it means breaking a pattern, not allowing my history to have power over my present?
- To live in the here and now?

How do you plan on executing this?

Do it daily.

The Addict (extremist)

At first, it feels like a blessing. A healthy diet, challenging workouts, and a fun supportive community. You feel great. You're in the best shape of your life. Yes, but if you're also a recovering addict or struggle with addictive behavior, you maneuver in extremes. You're all or nothing. This means you're buying CrossFit clothes, using CrossFit language in reference to things that have nothing to do with CrossFit, like your lunch. You're subscribing to blogs, watching CrossFit videos, checking your box's Leaderboard every two seconds. Suddenly CrossFit is your new addiction. You've developed a dependence on this activity despite the negative consequences associated with it. You may argue that there are no negative consequences associated with it. Are you putting other responsibilities aside for CrossFit? Are you spending beyond your means in membership, apparel, food, etc? Are you putting high expectations on your performance and internalizing them like the ex-athlete does? Are you using CrossFit as an escape from your marriage? Are you blurring boundaries with other members and coaches? Are you abusing CrossFit? If so, mental blocks will manifest. It's just a matter of time. Drama from the box, burn out, stress from home because you are never there (which leads to relationship problems), internal pressures to eat perfect and be the best, these will all get in the way of your CrossFit performance and experience.

The Person Who Lost 90 Pounds But Still Thinks He/She is Fat

You discovered CrossFit after losing "Subway Guy" weight. It happened fast and it changed your life. You love telling people how much weight you've lost just to see the expression on their face. But, deep inside, you still carry the false belief that you are overweight. This causes you to hide. You are afraid of judgment. You prefer to be invisible because that's what you're used to. That's how the world treated you. This knee jerk reaction becomes a mental block. You pull back instead of push through. It shows in your WODs.

Or you swing the complete other way and become an overachiever. You put on a cape and place an unrealistic amount of pressure on yourself. Your death grip resistance on not wanting to going back to the old you turns your cape into a noose. You place an unrealistic amount of pressure on yourself. (Note: Not wanting to go back to the old you can be a tool for strength but only if there are no false beliefs attached. In this case, there are false beliefs that make it a dangerous tool.)

The Short / Small Man Complex

If you're short or small, you know. The world has told you in some form, probably more than once, and you've been carrying it ever since. The false belief that you are lacking because of your size has turned your dial to survival mode and you have become funny. Or fast. Or both. This is wonderful. The world can use more funny, fast people. However, not if you are still in survival mode. You have a chip on your shoulder and a mindset that drives you to prove something, to compensate for what you believe you lack. This creates a space for that same unhealthy added pressure mentioned above.

The "I'm Too Old" Guy

You feel like the college kid at the high school party. Every time someone questions your performance or you don't do well, you blame your age. The false belief is that this is a young man's sport. Secretly you compete with them because if you can beat them, it means you're not old. Chasing this carrot creates unhealthy pressure. Again, you're setting yourself up for a fall and that drop is steep. Every time you drop, you internalize. And the record that plays in your head is that you are too old. This becomes a mental block. Your potential is hindered.

The Non-Athlete

My story.

The "I Don't Want to Get Too Big" Girl

This applies to both sexes, but I will focus on females because I see it in them the most. They don't want raging biceps and lats that make them look like flying squirrels. Their fear is that they will wake up one day looking like bodybuilders. I don't believe this is a size issue, I believe it's a masculine / feminine issue. If this is you, ask yourself what your beliefs are about what feminine and masculine looks like. How was that picture formed? Where did you learn it? Was it from an event? How someone treated you? Society's (the media's) view on beauty? Maybe a combination of all of these? Can CrossFit be a way to explore your beliefs on what is feminine and what is masculine? Can CrossFit be a way to redefine what that looks like? Can CrossFit be a way to take the power back so you don't define what is feminine by society's standards?

All the above archetypes have something in common. How we view ourselves, the false beliefs we posses, and the unhealthy pressures that build from that. You may or may not fall into any of these archetypes. But chances are, you do have false beliefs about yourself and these beliefs hold you back from your potential. No? Not even one?

Remember my definition of a mental block? Any thought or feeling that prevents us from our desired behavior and potential. If false beliefs fall under the feeling category (feeling about self), cognitive distortions are in the thought department. They are distorted thought patterns that convince us of something that isn't true. These thoughts sound rational and accurate but they actually keep us feeing bad about ourselves. They are mental blocks. Think of them as cousins of false beliefs.

Below is a list of some common cognitive distortions. Ask yourself if you relate to any of them.

Common Cognitive Distortions

Filtering

Taking the negative details and magnifying them while filtering out all positive aspects of a situation.

In the Box

- You just did Fran and got a PR but it wasn't the top time of the day. Instead of being happy about your new personal record, you are angry because you didn't come in first.

- Getting a great time on a WOD but beating yourself up because you couldn't RX it.

- Instead of seeing how far you've come, focusing on everything you still can't do.

Polarized Thinking (or "Black and White" Thinking)

Things are either "black" or "white." You are either perfect or you are a failure — there is no middle ground. You place people, usually yourself, or situations in "either/or" categories, with no shades of gray or allowing for the complexity of most people and situations. If your performance falls short of perfect, you see yourself as a total failure.

In the Box

- The coach says you've improved significantly but "you're still not fully locking out on your overhead squats". Instead of taking this information as progress / growth / encouragement, you take it as "I have failed again".

- You usually get within the top three times of the day. Today, you get fourth. Based on your performance on today's WOD, you believe that as you are not as good of a CrossFitter as the other three.

- If I don't get into Regionals, I don't want to CrossFit anymore.

Overgeneralization

Coming to a general conclusion based on a single incident or a single piece of evidence. If something bad happens only once, we expect it to happen over and over again. Seeing a single, unpleasant event as part of a never ending pattern of defeat.

In the Box

- You come in last once during a 5K so you believe you will always be last in every running WOD.

- You get a DNF on a certain WOD and believe you will always get a DNF on that particular WOD.

- Not qualifying for a local CrossFit competition causes you believe you will never qualify for any CrossFit competition.

Jumping to Conclusions

Without anyone saying so, believing that you know what others are feeling and why they act the way they do. In particular, determining how people are feeling toward us with no evidence. Simply put, to assume.

In the Box

- The coach doesn't give you the attention and encouragement she normally gives you during today's class, so you think she doesn't like you anymore.

- You don't get the same praise from this person as you do that person, so this person must be jealous of you and wants to see you fail.

- Your box didn't "Like" or comment on your WOD time you posted on their Facebook page. This must mean that they don't like or care about you.

Catastrophizing

The inability to foresee anything other than the worst possible outcome, however unlikely, or experiencing a situation as unbearable or impossible when it is just uncomfortable.

In the Box

- "It's a 45 minute AMMRAP. There's no way I can finish it. There's no way. I'll die."

- "If I do box jumps as fast as I can, I will fall and cut my shin. I saw it happen to someone once."

- "What if I drop a kettle bell on my face?"

Blaming

Holding other people responsible for our pain, or taking the other track and blaming ourselves for every problem.

In the Box

- Blaming the coach that programmed the WOD if we didn't do well or got injured during it.

- Blaming yourself for not being able to do something. This happens often when other members that have started around the same time as you have completed a task or goal. Double unders, muscle ups, and butterfly pull ups, for example.

- Blaming our parents for our poor eating habits.

Shoulds

Having a list of ironclad rules about how others and we should behave. We feel guilty when we violate these rules and angry when others break them.

In the Box

- The shoulds we place on ourselves. We should be at a certain weight. We should have a certain diet. We should lifting a certain weight. We should be a certain speed. We should come dressed a certain way. We should smell a certain way. We should have a certain attitude.

- Coaches placing shoulds on their clients, not because it's coming from a place of motivation, but rather the coaches own anger and frustration.

- Telling others what they should be trying to lift or do and getting angry or frustrated if they don't follow your shoulds.

Emotional Reasoning

Believing that what we feel must be true automatically. We assume that our unhealthy emotions reflect the way things really are — "I feel it, therefore it must be true."

In the Box

- I feel stupid and uncoordinated because I can't do double unders, therefore I am.

- I feel weak because I can't lift this. Therefore I am weak.

- I feel fat, therefore I am.

Fallacy of Change

Expecting other people to change to suit us for our own happiness. We need to change people because our hopes for happiness seem to depend entirely on them.

In the Box

I think many coaches struggle with this. Their worth depends on the change or results they see in their clients. Because of this cognitive distortion, they become angry, frustrated, and resentful if their clients don't meet their expectations.

We (members) do this with our friends by putting on our "coach" hat. We even do it with non-members when we desperately try to get our friends and family into CrossFit, even when they've told us over and over it's not for them.

Fighting Cognitive Distortions

Cognitive distortion patterns begin in childhood and can go unnoticed for years. They manifest in everything we do. They become part of who we are quite by habit. The first thing we need to do is be aware of them, to notice any of these distortions so that we can break our habits and begin to rewire ourselves.

Once you have noticed your negative thought pattern, reframe.

Filtering - Focusing on the negatives and filtering out all the positives.

The next time you feel yourself filtering (maybe you didn't get an expected PR, you came in last during a benchmark WOD, you couldn't do a handstand push up, or you didn't qualify for a local throw down), stop your thinking pattern. Focus on the positives and your accomplishments. Pull back. Look at the big picture. What PRs have you gotten recently?

When have you filtered recently? It doesn't have to be CrossFit related. It's about the thought process, not the content.

_____

_____

_____

REFRAME IT.

_____

_____

_____

_____

_____

_____

_____

_____

Polarized Thinking (Black and white thinking) - All or nothing thinking. Thinking in absolute terms. Win / fail.

There are very few situations that are absolute. When you hear "always / never / every", stop that thought. Instead, think of all times when these words were not true. Explore the grays and be comfortable with them. Accept and know that there is a middle ground and it's enough.

When was the most recent time you polarized your thinking? Describe it. What happened?

_____

_____

REFRAME IT.

_____

_____

_____

_____

_____

_____

_____

Overgeneralization - Taking a single negative experience and expecting it to forever be true.

We all have negative events that have happened during our lives. We hold on to those events. Or, more accurately, those events have a hold on us. The challenge is to know that we can create different outcomes in the future. Instead of stating "I didn't make it to Regionals this time so I probably won't make it ever", say and believe "I didn't make it this year, but I know what I need to work on. I'll work hard at that and make it next year". Remember that a single negative experience doesn't hold true forever. Every outcome is different. There are too many variables in life. There is no way to predict what's going to happen.

What was the last time you overgeneralized? Describe the situations / your thought process. Be specific.

_____

_____

_____

_____

_____

_____

_____

_____

_____

_____

_____

REFRAME IT.

_____

_____

_____

_____

_____

_____

_____

_____

_____

_____

_____

Catastrophizing - an irrational thought believing that something is far worse than it actually is, the kind of thing that happens when you're lying awake at three in the morning worried sick about the future and what's going to happen to you.

Catastrophic thinking proceeds like a chain. One "what if" leads to another until you're picturing yourself homeless. Or in this case, going back to a global gym. The key is to stop the chain, to short circuit it. To do this, write down each step in your catastrophic thoughts and challenge the plausibility of these events actually happening.

Describe the last time you catastrophized. Write it like a chain, one thought processing the next. Where do your thoughts end up?

_____

_____

_____

_____

_____

_____

_____

_____

REFRAME IT. (challenge the plausibility of these events actually happening)

_____

_____

Emotional Reasoning - a cognitive error that occurs when someone believes that what he or she is feeling is true regardless of the evidence.

Know your emotions. Notice what was going through your mind when the emotion appeared. What evidence supports the thought that produced the emotion? What's another way to look at the situation that is more rational and balanced? Consider your options. Make a choice.

When was the last time you experienced emotional reasoning? Describe it.

_____

_____

_____

_____

_____

_____

_____

REFRAME IT.

_____

_____

_____

Fallacy of Change - Expecting others to change in order for us to be happy.

You cannot change anyone. That is a fact. Swallow it. There is a brick wall behind that door so don't even open it. Thinking this way leaves you powerless, which causes anxiety and stress. In order to take that power back, focus solely on changing yourself.

When was the last time your happiness was dependent on someone else changing? Describe it.

_____

_____

_____

_____

_____

_____

_____

_____

_____

_____

_____

_____

REFRAME IT. (how can you change yourself
instead?)

_____

_____

_____

_____

_____

_____

_____

_____

_____

_____

_____

The goal is to train your brain. In order to do this, you must stop thoughts as you recognize them and reframe, over and over. The more you do this, the less impact your distortions will have. They will leave faster.

Double Standard

Many tend to treat others better than they do themselves. When our friend struggles with false beliefs or cognitive distortions, it's easy to see that those thoughts are not real. We even try to help them overcome those thoughts and beliefs. Step out of yourself and see it through their eyes. Then treat yourself as you would a friend. Imagine what you would say to them and say it to yourself.

Use Different Words

Sometimes changing words can make a huge impact. If you say, I "should" be able to hit a certain time or lift a certain weight, it creates negative feelings and thoughts inside you. There are expectations there and if you don't meet them, you internalize. This process can create a false belief / cognitive distortion. So replace any "shoulds" or "musts" or "oughts" with "woulds" or coulds" or "want tos". Instead of "I should be able to do that WOD under a certain time", you can say "It would be nice if I could do it in that time. But right now, I'm doing the best I possibly can". Changing the way you speak to yourself can take the pressure off.

CrossFit High School

The combination of CrossFit boxes opening on every block and the popularity of team competitions have amplified box spirit. It has strengthen communities and has built powerful bonds with it's members. But with strong athletic bonds and team competitions come rivalry. And with any rivalry, there is space for negativity - character assignation, rumors, judgement, etc. When CrossFit was in is infancy, spotting someone wearing a CrossFit t-shirt from a different box created an instant unity, a "we" connection. People in same fraternities from different chapters experience this same oneness. Now that CrossFit is booming and teams are forming within each box, box spirit is at an all time high. We support our box / team by wearing our box's logos on our shorts, socks, and head. We come to competitions sporting our box's colors, yelling, screaming, and cheering for our team. It makes sense. We have a fierce commitment to the place we sweat in daily. Today, if we see someone wearing a T-shirt from a different box, especially if that box "competes" with ours, we may feel animosity, envy, jealousy, or even hate. Competition becomes a crowbar. This process then eliminates what I believe makes CrossFit different than any other sport, the tremendous amount of sportsmanship for other athletes. There are very few sports where competitors go back and push / encourage their competition after they have won. There is enormous value in teams and in box spirit. I just vote we don't allow that to ruin the spirit of CrossFit because in that negative space, there is room for mental blocks.

Box Jumpers

We grow attached to our boxes. We establish relationships and build community. We eat, sweat, and share stories with each other. The box gives us support, encouragement, and a reason to be a better version of ourselves. We depend on our box. We have disagreements with our box. We get frustrated with our box. We forgive our box. We love our box. Our box becomes like a boyfriend / girlfriend. But like any relationship, we can also grow apart from our box. The spirit of the box might have changed or we may be seeking something different. Maybe the people we've started with are no longer there and we feel less connected?

Or maybe it's a financial thing. Whatever the reason, we may one day want to start seeing another box. It's important that we don't leave with residue. Like breaking up with your partner and bringing baggage into the next relationship, we must terminate the relationship in a healthy way. What does that look like? First, you have to ask yourself why you are leaving. Do you truly believe your box is not a good fit anymore or is this your way of running, hiding, pouting? If your exit is due to one bad experience, that is not enough to leave. You wouldn't break up with someone because of one fight, would you? You have invested a lot into your box and your presence, not only as an athlete but as a human being, is valuable. Your absence will effect the box (community). That's a fact. But if you've been there for a few years and feel you need a change, you have different goals or you're seeking a new community, that's fair. Just don't slip out. Don't just disappear. That is not fair to this box or the next one you join since you will be bringing your negative energy (baggage) into it. Think of it as leaving an expired relationship. Bring closure before you bail. Express / resolve with the staff, coaches, members so that you can leave with no residue. If not, you are risking your performance. Yes, your performance. The unresolved anger / frustration will become a mental block - any thought / behavior that gets in the way of your potential. It may be subconscious and you may not realize it until you're half way through a heavy lifting WOD in your new box and you find yourself furious, blaming the "ex" for not believing / supporting you. This is residue. Congratulations, you have a new mental block. Just like entering a new relationship, without a clean mindset, you will carry negative energy with you. Be responsible. Close this chapter before you open a new one. The dangling carrot. If you can do it, you are not only getting stronger physically but also emotionally / mental. You are becoming a better you, which is what CrossFit is all about, right?

Conclusion

CrossFitters talk about eating "clean". I believe it is just as important to think clean. This means making an effort to dissolve your false beliefs and cognitive distortions, to face your fears, accept your story, and to be the best version of yourself that you can be. If you are not on a path of doing these things, your mental and emotional diet is poor. If you believe CrossFit is 70, 80, 90 percent mental, how do you think your state will affect your game? If you want to maximize your potential, you must think clean.

Give

Your box is not a gym. It's a therapeutic community. You are rebuilding yourself through others and they are rebuilding themselves through you. This means we have a responsibility. We must work on our mental and emotional state, dissolve our false beliefs, and enter the box as the very best version of ourselves so that we can ignite change. Our focus should not just be our numbers but our community, our spirit, and the ripple we send with our story. CrossFit is not a workout regiment, but a potential movement for change. It only depends on your mindset.

Remember when I said I am just your average CrossFitter? That is a false belief. There is no such thing as an average CrossFitter. There is nothing average about us. We CrossFit because we posses courage. We seek improvement by challenging ourselves daily, staring fear in the face, and pushing ourselves harder than most. We are not CrossFitters because we breathe fire. We are CrossFitters because we believe in change and are determined to prove it.

Truth Five.

ABOUT ME

I am a licensed marriage family therapist with a public practice. I define my practice as "public" because I do everything online, including individual sessions, couples, and group work. I believe in using new media as therapeutic tools as well as a conduit to collect stories. If you would like to process with me, meet me at -

www.theangrytherapist.com

CPSIA information can be obtained at www.ICGtesting.com
Printed in the USA
LVOW01s2115160813

348285LV00023B/1137/P